How To Get The Most Out Of Your Massage

335 Great Massaging Tips

ADAM COLTON

Published by BizMove
www.bizmove.com

ISBN: 1979413274
ISBN- 978-1979413275

335 Great Massaging Tips

Have you ever wondered what it's like to give a massage at home? Is massage therapy something that interests you? Well, if you have answered yes to either of these questions, you may find the following tips of interest. There are so many ways you can give or get a massage which is why these tips were compiled with you in mind!

1. Petrissage is the best way to relieve stress and make pain disappear. This method requires you to use your fingertips and your thumb. Grab hold of a muscle and squeeze it for a few seconds before moving on to a different area. Go over the same areas several times until the pain disappears.

2. Oils such as sweet almond and olive oil are known for their healing properties. Oil is a better option than lotion or gel since it will be absorbed by the skin. Additionally, olive oil serves as a wonderful lubricant for the body.

3. In order to give a great massage, it's important that you carefully watch your subject. Pay close attention to facial expression and muscle tension. Practice

will make perfect as you explore their body. If they tense, you are applying too much pressure.

4. When using massage oil, before putting it on a person's back, place it into your hands first. If you place the oil directly onto your partner, the oil may be surprisingly cold and startle the person. That's not the kind of reaction you want from a massage. Instead place the oil first in your hands and warm the oil up by rubbing your hands together. This will make the oil the perfect temperature to use.

5. If you suffer from PMS each month with excessive water retention and cramping, there just might be some help for you. The power of massage has been shown to help reduce that unsightly water retention so that your pants will fit a little easier. It also can help relieve the pain that comes with cramps.

6. Discuss your problematic areas with your massage therapist. A massage's goal is to relax your muscles and target your problem areas. Therapists aren't psychics, so you have to guide them.

7. Try to save conversation for after the massage. You may love chatting with your massage therapist, but talking during the massage prevents you from ever relaxing fully. In fact, it may actually cause some muscles to tense up, making your therapist's job

even more difficult. Do speak up about your needs, however -- if the room's too cold, the music is too loud, or any other factor that prevents you from sinking deep into relaxation.

8. Speak up about potential medical issues. If you suffer from an illness that could be aggravated by a massage or if you are pregnant, say something. Your masseuse will be able to adjust their technique to give you a great massage that works around your ailment and keeps you safe.

9. If you have any medical conditions, such as you are pregnant, make sure that you let your massage therapist know. Some techniques may not be appropriate for your condition, so it is best to let the therapist know before starting. This will give him or her enough time to adjust techniques.

10.   This may be something you already know, but make sure you tip your massage therapist generously. It is not only the kind thing to do, but also earns the respect of your therapist if you plan on returning. Always show up on time for your massage because it not only shows you are serious, but you won't cut into someone else's massage time.

11.   If you feel as though your complexion is looking a little dull, or you are noticing little wrinkles

forming in places around your face, you do not have to run to the plastic surgeon! Giving yourself a daily face massage will promote blood flow to your skin, brightening it up and making those wrinkles virtually disappear.

12.   If you enjoy working out, you should try massaging your muscles before and after exercising. You should pummel your muscles with your fists to improve your circulation before working out and massage your muscles more gently after working out to speed up the recovery process. Make sure you stretch after massaging.

13.   Listen to your massage therapist and follow any professional directions they give you. They are the experts after all. As long as this person is being professional, trust that they know what is best. This includes any requests before and immediately following a massage. There may be things you need to do to make sure your muscles respond well.

14.   Doing eye massages can relieve tired and sore eyes. The main benefit of this massage is using warmth to relieve pain and strain. Begin this massage by rubbing your hands together vigorously. Do this until your hands start to feel warm. When hands are warm, cover each eye with a palm until the warmth goes away.

15.   When getting a massage, your actions will help you enjoy the massage more and receive maximum benefits from it. Practice deep breathing exercises while you are getting your massage. Breathe out when pressure is applied and breathe in when pressure is released. This will have an immeasurable impact on the relaxation of your massage.

16.   When getting up from a massage, do so slowly. Roll to your right side and sit up slowly. Ask your massage therapist for a hand if you need it. Do not stand too quickly or move around the room too suddenly. You might feel dizzy after a massage, and taking this approach can help you to avoid slips and falls.

17.   If you are on the giving end of a very beneficial massage, make sure to read the signs the recipient is showing. During a deep-tissue massage, the body responds to pressure and muscles will actually contract under your finger-tips. Ease up on the pressure when you approach bones and joints and be guided by the response you get!

18.   You should always make use of your thumbs when giving a massage. You have a lot of strength in your thumbs and can use these fingers to really

dig into the deeper tissues. Remember not to press too hard when massaging.

19.   If you are an athlete or have excessively hard workouts then having massages regularly is a good idea. Massages can loosen your muscles up before a game or exercise to help them from becoming injured. It can also help after strenuous exercise to help heal your muscles and keep them from stiffening up or becoming painful.

20.   Massage is great during pregnancy, but wait until after the first trimester. During the first trimester, your baby is in the earliest stages of development. Toxins released during a massage can harm the fetus or inhibit growth during this delicate period. Once you have reached 16 weeks, you should be all clear to enjoy a massage.

21.   Be certain to be on time or early at your masseuse's office. It is not difficult to lose track of the time. When this happens and you find yourself rushing in for your massage, it will take longer for you to relax during the massage. You want to be relaxing as you first get on the massage table.

22.   If you're going to get a massage, be sure to eat an extremely light meal before it. Eating a heavy meal before your massage could make you

uncomfortable and prevent you from enjoying your experience. Eat a light, nutritious meal before your massage to allow yourself to enjoy every moment of the massage.

23. If a person wants a deeper massage, be careful on how much oil, you use. Yes, oil feels great on a person's back and causes less friction, but the latter is the problem for deeper tissue massage. Without that friction, you won't be able to offer a deep massage, as your hands will constantly slide. Minimize this issue by using just enough oil for the massage to be comfortable, but not so much that you lose all friction.

24. If you notice knots in the back while you are giving a massage, you can kneed them out with some pressure from your fists. Simply get your fists into a ball and work them over the knotted spot for a few minutes. Apply more pressure if the knots are deeper, as long as the recipient remains comfortable.

25. A foot massage can be used for more than tired, achy feet. You can search online and find foot maps that show which area of the foot can be massaged to experience relief from a myriad of symptoms throughout your body. For example, pressing on

the big toe is known to relieve sinus pain and pressure.

26.   The magnitude of pressure used when you are getting a massage is significant for various goals. If someone's muscles are knotted, use slow-moving pressure to ease the tension. Even if you just keep constant pressure on the knot, you will feel the release of tension. This is the main idea behind deep tissue massage.

27.   Asian massages are known to help relax the body. One not-so-common, but very relaxing Asian massage is called the Indonesian-Javanese massage. With this method, the therapist will use both their hands and knuckles to get so deep into the skin. This will help your muscles relax if they were tense.

28.   Be aware that it may take awhile before you are an expert masseuse. Begin by providing massages for people you know, and ask them to provide feedback. Practice on people who will give you accurate feedback.

29.   Help the massage therapist by relaxing your body. Avoid trying to "help" by tensing certain muscles or areas. The massage therapist is well-educated in various ways to maneuver your body parts to achieve the best results from massage, but

their work is hindered if you can't relax. Try doing some deep breathing and practice just letting go and trusting the therapist to do a great job.

30.   If you need help with stress or pain, you should get a massage from a professional. Asking someone you know to give you a massage can be helpful but keep in mind that a trained professional will be able to use technique your friend or relative does not know about.

31.   It's possible to give yourself a great foot massage using an easy strategy that athletes use. Just use a tennis ball or a golf ball to massage the sole of your foot. Shift your feet back and forth and to and fro. Concentrate on the arch area of your foot which is more sensitive.

32.   Incredibly, there is a type of massage everyone can do after eating their meal. Place both palms of your hands on your stomach, and move them both in a circular fashion. This helps to promote digestion because this is how food moves though the intestines.

33.   If you are giving a deep tissue massage, incorporate your elbows into it. This may feel uncomfortable at first for the person you are massaging, but is a fantastic way of spreading out

the muscle and causing a very pleasurable sensation. Never push too hard though, as this will then feel uncomfortable.

34.   Even though there are many wonderful benefits to having a massage, if you have a lot of health problems or an injury you should talk to your doctor first. What you might think is a harmless massage could end up causing a condition to worsen such as a blood clot.

35.   You should have an open mind when getting a massage. If you are getting a massage for the first time, you might find the whole process a bit unusual. Don't let this discourage you from relaxing and having an enjoyable time. Just calm down and allow the masseuse to do what they do best.

36.   If you are an athlete or have excessively hard workouts then having massages regularly is a good idea. Massages can loosen your muscles up before a game or exercise to help them from becoming injured. It can also help after strenuous exercise to help heal your muscles and keep them from stiffening up or becoming painful.

37.   Feeling a little blue? Go get a massage! The health benefits of massage are numerous, and studies have shown that one of the benefits of

massage is elevated serotonin. Serotonin is a neurochemical that makes us feel happy, yet lack of sleep, hormone fluctuations, gloomy weather and poor diets can lower your body's natural serotonin stores.

38.   Try to get a good massage a couple times per week. Your overall health and your mood will improve if you are able to make massage a regular part of your routine. Massages allow you to relax and let go of the stress and tension you have been carrying around with you. If possible, try having a massage no less than twice a week.

39.   It is always best to stay with a licensed massage therapist when having a massage. A therapist with a license has had training and can understand your needs better. Hiring a professional will guarantee a specific professionalism advocated by the person's industry.

40.   Stretch before you go to get a message. This will help to loosen you up just a little bit before hand so that your massage therapist can quickly locate any problem areas that you might have. If you have extreme pain you may not want to do this, otherwise it is a good idea.

41.   Lubrication is important when giving a massage. The best lubricants will allow your hands to glide across the body. Oils work well as do many lotions. Try out a few different kinds and see which works best. You want a lotion that will not require reapplication causing breaks during the massage.

42.   A foot massage can be used for more than tired, achy feet. You can search online and find foot maps that show which area of the foot can be massaged to experience relief from a myriad of symptoms throughout your body. For example, pressing on the big toe is known to relieve sinus pain and pressure.

43.   Try using your fists to give a good massage. Gently thump on the area that is painful or tense after warming the muscles with a more gentler techniques. Thumping is excellent for circulation and will cause the entire muscle to relax almost instantly. Avoid using this technique on someone who has to take blood thinners to prevent bruising.

44.   Don't swear off using a massage therapist of the opposite sex. You may initially be weird about it, but get over it! Men may have the height and strength you need to work out the kinks from a really bad back, and women may have the relaxed

touch you need to de-stress. Be open to whoever may best fit your current need.

45.   Before beginning your massage, discuss pressure with your massage therapist. Some people like massages that are very deep with a hard intensity. Others prefer a lighter touch or even Reiki style massages where touch is not necessary. If you let your therapist know what works for you, they can adjust the massage to meet your individual needs.

46.   Engage in a dialogue when you are giving your massage. This is important as you not only want to know if you are doing things right, but if the person is comfortable or not. This is crucial to know if you are applying pressure, as you do not want to hurt them or have them feel nothing at all.

47.   Many ailments can be alleviated with regular visits to a massage parlor. From debilitating conditions like Fibromyalgia to simple stress, a massage can do wonders for both mind and body. Consider this alternative to more medication or tolerating more pain and discomfort. Ask your doctor if a healthy massage can help you out!

48.   If you often experience back pain, you should consider investing in a vibrating massaging pad. Some pads even have an option that allows you to

apply heat to your muscles. Compare different products before you purchase on and choose one with different speeds so you can easily adjust it in function of your needs.

49.   Try playing soft music while giving a massage. This music can help to soothe and relax the individual receiving your massage. That relieves tension in sore muscles. You will very likely see improved benefits as tightened muscles gradually get looser.

50.   You do not have to get totally naked during a massage if you do not feel comfortable with that. You can strip down to your undergarments and have the masseuse cover you up with a towel. This way you can get your entire body massaged without feeling the least bit awkward.

51.   If you are planning on giving your partner a massage, do not be too upset if they are not willing to return the favor immediately. If you do the job right, your partner should be so relaxed, they will not want to give a massage right after. Plan on trading off and taking turns in giving and receiving of massages.

52.   Seek to have your massages done professionally. While it may be easier to ask for one from your

spouse, you are certainly risking injury. If someone is not educated in how to properly give a massage. They can easily cause a muscle to be pulled or even something far worse.

53.   Change your mindset about massage. Instead of thinking of it as a luxury, think of massage as a therapeutic approach to health. Research shows that massage can lower levels of the stress hormone cortisol, as well as lessening asthma symptoms in children. Additionally, those tension headaches are no match for the hands of a skilled massage therapist.

54.   Try getting a therapeutic massage. There has been proof that this type of massage can lower stress levels, help get rid of tension headaches caused by contracting muscles in the face, neck and head, and better the breathing of asthmatic children. It's believed that is type of massage is so successful due to people believing in it so much, which creates a powerful mind and body connection.

55.   You should try different techniques when giving a massage. Use your hands and fingers to rub, apply pressure or even give gentle taps. Use the tip of your fingers if you need precision, for instance to relax a tense muscle. You could also try covering as

much surface as possible by using the palm of your hands to apply pressure.

56.   When giving a massage, it is very important that you use oil or lotion. Massage oils can increase the movements of the soft tissue. Using oil will minimize the pinching and tugging feel on the skin. Massage oils come in all different varieties. They include aromatherapy and provide lubrication and nutrients.

57.   If you have recently contracted the flu, a massage may help alleviate the pain and stiffness generally associated with the flu. For the best relief, gently rub warmed lotion over your entire body using a circular motion. This will not only alleviate aches, but it will also help re-hydrate your skin.

58.   Like acupuncture, Japanese Shiatsu massage works on the pressure points. Instead of using needles, the Shiatsu practitioner applies fingertip pressure. This will tap into the different pressure points on your body to stimulate pleasure. The goal of Shiatsu massage is to increase one's well being and energy level.

59.   Try using your fists to give a good massage. Gently thump on the area that is painful or tense after warming the muscles with a more gentler

techniques. Thumping is excellent for circulation and will cause the entire muscle to relax almost instantly. Avoid using this technique on someone who has to take blood thinners to prevent bruising.

60.   There are a few secrets to giving a fantastic massage and they involve things you don't do. Always be careful to not pull their hair. Body hair is included in this. Be careful of pressure on their bones. Learn to be gentle when you need to be and hard when required.

61.   Before you get a massage, talk with the therapist about any health problems you have. You will particularly want to inform the masseuse if you are expecting a baby. This information will assist the massage therapist in tailoring the massage to your specific needs. You might make things worse if you do not know what you are doing.

62.   Surprising, a certain massage should be used by all people when done eating. It involves putting your hands on you belly and moving them around. This helps you with proper digestion.

63.   Doing eye massages can relieve tired and sore eyes. The main benefit of this massage is using warmth to relieve pain and strain. Begin this massage by rubbing your hands together vigorously.

Do this until your hands start to feel warm. When hands are warm, cover each eye with a palm until the warmth goes away.

64.   If your partner needs a deep massage, use your body weight to help. Massaging strictly with your hands can get exhausting very fast, making the massage less enjoyable for the both of you. When you put some weight into it, it is easier to go deeper and provide a longer massage experience.

65.   When you go for your massage, you are paying good money for a relaxing experience. Do not ruin your massage by not using the restroom before you begin. The best massages are continuous from 45 minutes to an hour. If you have to take a break in the middle of the massage for a restroom break, you are not going to be fully relaxed at the end of your session.

66.   Let's be honest, your masseuse isn't interested in rubbing your dirty feet. Take a shower and wash every inch before you arrive to your appointment. Your masseuse will not only thank you, but you will also prevent smelling your own aroma while being massaged.

67.   It can be extremely beneficial to get regular prenatal massages if you are pregnant. These

massages are specially designed to ease the unique aches and pains associated with pregnancy, and can benefit your baby as well. It has been said that developing babies will grow quicker in those women who receive regular prenatal massages.

68.   Know your options before getting a massage. There are many different techniques and some of these methods may not work well with your body or any injuries you have. Each has its own pros and cons.

69.   Many ailments can be alleviated with regular visits to a massage parlor. From debilitating conditions like Fibromyalgia to simple stress, a massage can do wonders for both mind and body. Consider this alternative to more medication or tolerating more pain and discomfort. Ask your doctor if a healthy massage can help you out!

70.   A massage can help your entire body feel better. If your back hurts chronically, or other stress issues are bothering you, get regular massages. See if someone you know can perform the service for you, or locate a professional therapist in your area.

71.   Start your massage at the top of the back. This is important as there are a lot of muscles and knots tied up in this area. This technique will help you to

soothe the person you are massaging and serves as a great bridge to the other areas of the body.

72.	It is important that you arrive on time, or better yet, early for your massage. You can easily be lost in time. If you have to rush or get there late, you will find it hard to relax and enjoy your massage. It is always best to be totally relaxed by the time you stretch out.

73.	If you experience stress or other negative emotions, you should try massaging specific points of your body. Target your nerve endings to get your body to relax. Sensitive nerve endings are located along your spine, the top of your head and in different parts of your face. You should try gently tapping on the top of your head, your forehead, cheeks and chin before taking a deep breath.

74.	Your massage therapist needs to be capable to get to your skin in order to do the massage, so you need to be prepared to disrobe. You will be able to do this in the room alone, and you can leave on your underwear. Once you are undressed and face down on the massage table under a sheet, then the therapist will return to the room.

75.	If you will be getting a massage to have some stress relieved, go with an aromatherapy massage.

Along with a massage, the therapist will use essential oils on your capillaries in order to relax the body. Most of these oils come from flowers, roots, and herbs and are completely safe.

76.   If you suffer from PMS each month with excessive water retention and cramping, there just might be some help for you. The power of massage has been shown to help reduce that unsightly water retention so that your pants will fit a little easier. It also can help relieve the pain that comes with cramps.

77.   There is no real dress code when you decide to go out and get a massage. If you are concerned about dressing appropriate, speak with the spa or your message therapist beforehand. By addressing clothing concerns, you can ensure that you won't feel embarrassed or uncomfortable during your massage. If there is an area you also don't want massaged like your behind, tell the therapist before starting.

78.   If you are a woman, don't swear off men massage therapists. Since most women are modest, they often feel uncomfortable in front of a male massage therapist. However, some women have reported that the best massage they have gotten in a long time is from a male massage therapist.

Whatever your decision, don't just base it on the sex of the massage therapist.

79.   Sports massage is a tool many athletes use today. Even if you are an amateur at exercise, sports massage can benefit you. These massages help increase stamina and strength, over time.

80.   Prior to getting a massage, inform your massage therapist of all the problem areas you have. If you don't you may end up wasting half of your massage time on areas that need a lot less work to feel good! This communication will give your therapist a plan of action for the limited time there is available.

81.   The goal of any massage is to make your partner feel good and relaxed. The massage will help with this, but the environment will also play a part in it as well. Set the mood and have some nice scents like candles or potpourri fill the air. Furthermore, a good massage table to make your partner comfortable will help tremendously.

82.   Try using your fists to give a good massage. Gently thump on the area that is painful or tense after warming the muscles with a more gentler techniques. Thumping is excellent for circulation and will cause the entire muscle to relax almost

instantly. Avoid using this technique on someone who has to take blood thinners to prevent bruising.

83.   Be on time, or a little early. Besides being good etiquette, being punctual can actually help your massage be effective. When you are running late, you are usually in a frenzied state, increasing stress levels and putting your body on edge. In a massage, this means it will take you longer to unwind and you may not get all of the benefits of a relaxing rub down.

84.   A great massage technique for reliving shoulder pressure is providing yourself with a bear hug. To do this, put the right hand on the left shoulder and the left hand on the right shoulder. Tightly press on each shoulder and release. Do this three times. Finally, begin to work your hands down your arms squeezing and then letting go until you get to your wrists.

85.   When you are stumped for what to give as a Christmas or birthday present, consider buying a coupon for a healthy massage! Everybody loves the soothing and relaxing benefits of a deep tissue massage and who couldn't use the extra pampering? Especially for the person who has everything, the gift of massage is perfect!

86.   A good way to eliminate stress and pain is by getting a massage. If your back hurts chronically, or other stress issues are bothering you, get regular massages. See if someone you know can perform the service for you, or locate a professional therapist in your area.

87.   Everyone is different, so make sure to switch up your techniques when giving massages. If there isn't a good response when you're massaging someone, make sure that you move from that area. Be mindful about your subjects' feedback during the massage.

88.   Keep the room at a good temperature throughout the entire massage. If you are giving a massage during the winter, try to have the heat on so that things are not uncomfortable. On the other hand, if it is very hot outside, keep the air conditioning on at a reasonable level.

89.   Make sure the person you give a massage to is comfortably installed. Ideally, you should use a massage table or at least a comfortable mat. If you do not have this equipment, have the person lay down on a comfortable couch or a supportive mattress. Make sure their head is properly supported.

90.   The pressure you apply during a massage depends on your goals. If you are working on someone with lots of tough knots, using pressure slowly will cut the tension. Don't overdo it though. This is the basic principle behind a deep tissue massage.

91.   If your child is suffering from colic, a gentle massage may alleviate some of their suffering. Slightly warm some lavender baby lotion and gently massage your infants back, legs, hands and feet. This will help relax your child making them less fussy if they are suffering from stomach cramps caused by colic.

92.   When you're stressed out or feeling emotional, aromatherapy massage is for you. The therapist will use essential oils while massaging your skin. They know exactly which oils will give you energy, relax you or help to bust stress. Lavender is frequently used to calm your mind and body, allowing you some peace.

93.   Tell your therapist where your problems lie. Massages are supposed to relax muscles and target the problem areas. Your therapist does not know you, which is why you need to tell him or her about your problems. They will be able to help you out best.

94.   If you are getting a full body massage, always ask to take a shower or at least wash your feet prior to beginning the massage. You can hold a lot of dirt and bacteria on places like your feet and hands, and you do not want your massage therapist massaging those areas first and then placing their hands on your face for further massage.

95.   What should one use for a self-massage? Whatever you can use! If you're massaging a knot out of your thigh, why not use your elbow? Is your neck sore? Fingers will do, but you can also buy a massaging neck roller. Try out different items and body parts and see what works for you.

96.   Try using your fists to give a good massage. Gently thump on the area that is painful or tense after warming the muscles with a more gentler techniques. Thumping is excellent for circulation and will cause the entire muscle to relax almost instantly. Avoid using this technique on someone who has to take blood thinners to prevent bruising.

97.   Do not neglect the hands and feet when you massage someone. These sensitive areas can make a massage very enjoyable. When you are massaging these areas, try to be as firm as possible to loosen up the muscles.

98.   How much should you tip a masseuse? If you're at a hotel or a local spa, 20% is pretty standard. If they work from home, each therapist will typically set their own policies, but 20% is fair. If they work in a massage clinic, ask them for their rules - some will include the tip in the price.

99.   When getting a massage, you need to fully relax as the therapist moves your body and joints. You do not need to try to help the therapist move your limbs and body. Think of it as being a puppet, with the therapist moving your body as they want and you just along for the ride.

100.   Those who like the practice of giving massages might want a license in massage therapy. It only takes a few months to get your license, and it should serve you well financially. You have the option of working for a massage clinic or starting your own home business.

101.   When you are giving a massage, the atmosphere you provide will do wonders for your partner. Try using soft music in the background to relax your partner. Diffuser oils and candles will relax your partners senses and make them feel at ease. Also using low or soft lighting will help your partner relax and get into the mood for a great massage.

102.   Why is it that you think a massage will help you?
Did you get involved in an auto accident? Does
your back hurt? Do you just want to relax? The
reason you are looking for a massage therapist can
be many, but make sure you choose the correct
therapist for you.

103.   You may already know that it is customary to tip
your masseuse. If you are new to this, tipping 15%
to 20% is customary. The only time you shouldn't
think about tipping is if you are getting physical
therapy treatments at a medical facility. Never hand
your masseuse a wad of cash, leave it at the front
desk with the clerk.

104.   One great massage technique that you can do
for your partner is called raking. Raking means that
you spread your hands out, and using your
fingertips, you rake up one side of the back right by
the spine while you rake downward on the other
side with your other hand.

105.   Hydrate yourself after receiving a massage. Your
muscles will release a lot of toxins while they are
massaged, and you might experience stress if you do
not purify your body from these toxins. Drink a lot
of water before and after your massage and be very

careful about your hydration if you get massages regularly.

106.   Use your thumbs when massaging. They are very handy little tools that help stimulate muscles. Be careful not to dig your thumbs into their muscle, though.

107.   Massage is great during pregnancy, but wait until after the first trimester. During the first trimester, your baby is in the earliest stages of development. Toxins released during a massage can harm the fetus or inhibit growth during this delicate period. Once you have reached 16 weeks, you should be all clear to enjoy a massage.

108.   You may have gotten some stretch marks from weight gain and loss or from pregnancy. Perhaps you have made a lot of attempts to rid yourself of them. Try massaging your problem spots with coco butter. When you apply the massage, the tissues respond by regenerating. This will reduce the marks over time.

109.   If your child suffers from asthma, consider massage. Massage has been proven to help breathing in asthmatic children due to the relaxing benefits it offers. A child's massage should be done with a gentle touch and only for a limited period of

time. Try this in the evening and help your child to also enjoy a good night's rest.

110.   Don't be afraid of appearing rude, ask any questions you have during your massage. There are no stupid questions, and your massage therapist should be happy to answer them. They just want you to be as comfortable as you can be, so be sure that you're getting any information that you need.

111.   Trigger-point therapy, also called neuromuscular therapy, involves the application of pressure to specific spots identified as trigger points. Tight knots often form in specific areas of irritated muscle tissue. Left untreated, these knots can lead to pain in around the area. Pressure applied to these areas cause the muscles to relax so the pain is relieved.

112.   The Japanese love to engage in a form of massage called shiatsu. This uses the pressure from the masseuse's fingers pressed in a rhythm on your acupuncture meridians. The pressure is applied for a few to many seconds, boosting energy flow and returning the body to balance. It doesn't leave you sore, either!

113.   Extend the benefits of your massage by taking things easy for the rest of the day. Allow your mind

and body to stay in the relaxed zone by practicing deep breathing throughout the day whenever you feel the tension returning. Plan a low-key, relaxing dinner followed by a warm bath, then get into bed early and curl up for a nice, restorative night of sleep

114.   There is a helpful massage that helps to relieve sinus pressure and congestion. To do this massage, begin by placing your fingers right above your nose and pressing down. Be sure you are rubbing outward. Next, put your fingers under your eyes, moving down and rubbing out. Massage the cheekbones with your thumbs and then put your thumbs on your temples, moving in small circles.

115.   Never get a massage if your doctor advises against it. This may seem obvious, but often, people will get a massage because they feel that it will help soothe them and make them feel better. If you have muscle tears, this could actually make them worse with constant pressure on your body.

116.   Consider why you want to get a massage. Have you been injured in an accident? Do you feel back pain constantly? Or are you looking for a healthy way to unwind and relax? Knowing the reason for your visit to a massage therapist is important in order to choose the one that suits you best.

117. Before and after you exercise, you should give your body a good massage. Before you exercise, use your fists in a pummeling motion to stimulate blood flow to your arms and legs. After you exercise, rub your muscles with your fist or palm. Move along your heart's direction. This helps to speed up your recovery and aids in waste removal.

118. After you get a massage, drink some water. Since massage works to detoxify your body, water is needed to flush the system. Try to stay away from soda or fruit drinks as they do not put anything good in your body. You will quickly feel stressed again if you do not get rid of these toxins.

119. You can give yourself a great foot massage by rubbing your heel and progressing toward your toes. Press firmly with the heel of the hand. Begin by massaging your toes with your fingers and thumb. Then, massage the top side of your foot, starting from your toes to your ankle After this first run through, keep doing the deep massage utilizing your thumb across your foot's bottom.

120. You do not have to get totally naked during a massage if you do not feel comfortable with that. You can strip down to your undergarments and have the masseuse cover you up with a towel. This

way you can get your entire body massaged without feeling the least bit awkward.

121.   If you are an athlete or have excessively hard workouts then having massages regularly is a good idea. Massages can loosen your muscles up before a game or exercise to help them from becoming injured. It can also help after strenuous exercise to help heal your muscles and keep them from stiffening up or becoming painful.

122.   When giving a massage, do not forget to focus some attention on the neck and shoulders. While much attention is paid to the back during a massage, the neck and shoulders can hold tension and stress too. Spending some time massaging them offers a lot of relief and can improve the massage experience.

123.   If you experience stress or other negative emotions, you should try massaging specific points of your body. Target your nerve endings to get your body to relax. Sensitive nerve endings are located along your spine, the top of your head and in different parts of your face. You should try gently tapping on the top of your head, your forehead, cheeks and chin before taking a deep breath.

124.   In order to give a great massage, it's important that you carefully watch your subject. You need to see how their muscles tighten and also observe their facial expressions. It takes practice, but over time you will be able to read their body with your hands. Understand that when your client is tense, you will need to ease up a bit.

125.   You can give yourself a hand massage by using a pencil with an eraser. Use the pencil eraser to press into the fleshy areas of your hand, paying particular attention to the thumb pad. Move the eraser in a circular motion around your hand maximizing the pressure if it is necessary.

126.   Hydrate, hydrate. A massage loosens lymph fluid, lactic acid and other toxins from your soft tissues. This is part of what makes your muscles feel so nice afterward. However, if you are dehydrated, there is no way for these toxins to leave your system. This could leave you feeling sore and slightly nauseated after your massage, which defeats the whole effort and wastes money. So, make sure you drink up!

127.   Be on time, or a little early. Besides being good etiquette, being punctual can actually help your massage be effective. When you are running late, you are usually in a frenzied state, increasing stress

levels and putting your body on edge. In a massage, this means it will take you longer to unwind and you may not get all of the benefits of a relaxing rub down.

128.   If you are going to be giving a massage, make sure that you are using lubricant. Lubricant can be any form of lotion or even therapeutic oils. Whichever you choose, make sure that it is appropriate for the recipient of the massage. Lubricants can help you glide across the body without disturbing the rhythmic movements.

129.   If you like gentle massages, request a Swedish massage. This type of massage uses long, gentle strokes. It has been described as the most relaxing type of massage available. This massage gently massages the superficial layers of muscle tissue resulting in relaxation and peace of mind. This type of massage is great for those who are new to massage therapy.

130.   Before massaging the back, make sure that the massage oil is warm. Cold oil applied directly to the skin is not pleasant and does not get the massage experience off on the right foot. It is better to put some oil on your hands, then spend a bit of time rubbing them together. Friction will provide the heat needed for the oil to reach a good temperature.

131. Eat some food about 30 minutes prior to a massage, but don't eat too much! You don't want to feel bloated for the experience. You want just enough food that you feel relaxed. If you go in hungry, you'll be that much more stressed for the entire time period of the massage.

132. Try not to go to a massage appointment with a full stomach. It is better to have eaten about half an hour before your appointment. A massage requires that you lay on your stomach for an extended period of time, and this can be very uncomfortable if your belly is too full.

133. After you eat, rub your stomach. Really! It's the truth! This helps you practice healthy digestion. To do this, place your palms on your abdomen and gently rub it in a clockwise circle. Because this tracks the path of your intestines, the digestive process will be aided.

134. Make sure your hands have been warmed prior to giving a massage. Hands that are cold don't feel good on someone's body, and they may make the person getting the massage more tense. Rub your hands with oil to help heat them up before a massage.

135.   If you are massaging your dog, understand that you should not be too forceful. This could hurt your dog. Pay attention to the body language of your pet. If he does not seem to enjoy the massage, stop doing it.

136.   When your massage is over with, drink an eight ounce glass of water. Water will help flush out toxins that were released during the massage. Water is great for the post-massage hours, and other beverages simply will not do. You will quickly feel stressed again if you do not get rid of these toxins.

137.   If you have a wound that is beginning to heal, massaging around that area will help it to heal even faster. Massage increases the amount of blood that is flowing to that area of your body. So, by massaging that area you are providing it with new blood to promote healing. This can also help to reduce scars.

138.   The speed of your hands is important for the kind of massage you are trying to give. If you are looking for a massage to relax your partner, go for slow strokes. If you are looking to work out tired muscles that have been over exerted, faster strokes work better.

139.   If you suffer from sinus pressure, use massage to help. A simple and quick massage under your brow line can help to clear your sinuses and make breathing much easier. Just use your fingers to massage gently over the eyes and across the bridge of your nose. This only takes minutes, and it can offer you a lot of relief.

140.   The magnitude of pressure used when you are getting a massage is significant for various goals. When muscles are tense, more pressure is needed. Even if you maintain constant pressure on your knots, the tension will ease. This is a fundamental part of all deep tissue massages.

141.   It is always helpful if you ask your massage client if they wouldn't mind shaving a day or two prior to the massage. This helps provide a smooth surface, specifically if you're using oil. This allows your hands to freely flow, resulting in a better massage.

142.   If you have a favorite fragrance of massage oil, bring it to your next massage. More than likely, the therapist will be willing to use it. Sometimes they may have a preference for oils of a certain type, but it is definitely worth asking to see if they are willing to use your favorite.

143.   The feet are an often overlooked area that needs to be massaged. There are many pressure points in the feet that can relax the body as a whole and give the entire body a sense of well being. Focus on one foot at a time and use as much pressure as your partner will allow.

144.   When you make the decision to get massage regularly, form a rapport with the massage therapist. If you trust your masseuse, you will have a more relaxing experience. To feel more secure, try chatting with your massage therapist before beginning your massage.

145.   Do not hesitate to talk to your doctor about massages. If you deal with back pains or muscle pains on a regular basis, ask your doctor if massages would be a good solution. Your doctor should be able to recommend a good massage clinic in your area and even write you a prescription.

146.   Athletes know about a sports massage. People who like exercising in an amateur sort of way can also benefit. These massages weren't designed to get rid of stress or to cause relaxation; they were made to make the body stronger to fight off injuries.

147.   Don't be intimidated about speaking up when you get a massage. Alert her to any specific area you

would like to focus on. If she does not rub hard enough to break up your deep knots, it is important that you speak up.

148.   When you go for your massage, you are paying good money for a relaxing experience. Do not ruin your massage by not using the restroom before you begin. The best massages are continuous from 45 minutes to an hour. If you have to take a break in the middle of the massage for a restroom break, you are not going to be fully relaxed at the end of your session.

149.   Do you have a cold? You can relieve sinus pressure by massaging your face gently. Massage your forehead and temples and apply gentle pressure around your nose and eyes. Repeat this process throughout the day until the pressure is gone. This technique is useful to relieve headaches and stress too.

150.   If you are unsure of which massage therapist to see in your area, ask your family members and coworkers. Referrals are crucial. While they don't ensure that you will get a great therapist, they do increase your odds tremendously. After you get a few names, do your own research to see which person you think best fits your needs.

151.   Wear loose fitting clothing to your massage. Your masseuse will ask you to disrobe down to the level of your comfort, and so the last thing you want to do is struggle with multiple layers or tight clothing as you get ready for your massage! Many people wear workout clothing when they get a massage.

152.   It's still possible to get a massage, regardless of how little money you have. Find a school in your area that offers massage therapy classes and see if they have a clinic. You can get discounted massages at these times.

153.   Massage therapy will help you heal quickly. You can benefit immensely from massage therapy if you have certain conditions that cause you pain. Massage is much healthier than certain types of drugs.

154.   If you plan to give a massage, ensure the atmosphere is right. Keep the air at room temperature and avoid any drafty windows or doors. In the background, play some easy listening music and light scented candles to really set the tone. Once the room is ready, get down to work!

155.   Ask you friends who they use for their massages. It can be hard to find a massage therapist

that you are comfortable with, but knowing that someone you know uses and trusts them you will feel that much better about it. Ask as many people as you can before you decide on one to try.

156.   When giving a massage, make sure that you use the right amount of pressure. It is a delicate balance between using too much pressure and not enough. Take some time to practice. Ask the person you are giving the massage to if you are using too much or too little. Their feedback should dictate the amount of pressure you use.

157.   Put your thinking on hold. One of the most difficult, yet essential elements of getting the most out of a massage is relaxing your mental state. Try to start doing some deep breathing while the therapist is setting up. Imagine that, with every inhale, you gather all the nagging and stressful thoughts in your head. On the exhale, envision blowing all of these thoughts out into space, gone forever. Keep repeating until you feel yourself relaxing.

158.   When you are giving a massage, try to have the person you are massaging in as few articles of clothing as possible. If they are uncomfortable, they can wear a towel to feel more secure at all times.

Having areas of the body exposed is not only soothing, but it also facilitates your job.

159. When you decide to get a massage, make sure you are communicating with your massage therapist. If you have any massage preferences, make sure you tell him or her when entering the room and before starting. If during the massage you are feeling pain or experiencing numbness, make sure you let your therapist know by speaking up.

160. A Shiatsu massage is very similar to an acupuncture session except the therapist uses fingers instead of needles. This will tap into the different pressure points on your body to stimulate pleasure. These particular massages have a goal of increasing energy and well being.

161. You can use a method that is touted by athletes to massage your feet. Message your feet by rolling over a tennis or golf ball. Do this over your full foot for maximum results. Spend more time on the arch since this area is more sensitive.

162. The legs are very important when giving a massage. Many of the largest muscles in the body are in the legs, and these are often the most used. Be responsive to your partner when massaging their legs and try to encompass the entire muscle group.

Start up high around the butt and work your way down to the ankles.

163.   When giving a massage to someone, you need to be careful about the amount of pressure you are putting in them. Applying too much pressure could cause damage to their nerves, joints and muscles. Also, you should be massaging toward the heart, as applying the wrong way could cause damage to veins.

164.   Finding the right therapist is very important when it comes to massages. You do not want to visit an inexperienced or inept therapist who may cause you more harm than good. Ask friends or family if they know of a good one in your area or look on the Internet for reviews.

165.   If you have a spot which hurts frequently, give it a massage once per day. This will help loosen it up and hopefully your pain will not return. Over time, you may find that it is already loose when you start to rub it, so you can reduce the frequency of massage.

166.   Sit down quietly for a couple minutes following a massage. A massage is a bit of a workout for your muscles. If you get up too quickly, your body may not respond well. In fact, you might even feel ill or

faint. Before you stand upright, breathe deeply and readjust slowly.

167.   When you decide to get a massage, make sure that you are relaxing your thoughts. It can be easy to feel nervous, especially if it's your first time. Most professional spas usually have relaxing music playing. If you hear the music, channel your thoughts into paying attention to the individual notes. This can help you relax in your tense moments.

168.   Is there a specific reason you are in need of a massage? Did you happen to be in an incident that involved an automobile crash? Do you suffer from back pain? Or do you just want to de-stress and relax? Knowing why you are having a message can help you choose the right professional for your needs.

169.   You do not need tons of money to receive a massage. Go to a local massage school and see when they've got their clinic. This discounted rate can save you a lot of money if you want to incorporate massages into your regimen.

170.   You want to make sure that you go to a reputable place that has professional staff members who are trained in the art of massage. Ask your

friends who have gotten massages before for their recommendations, and do some internet research to find reviews of good places in your area.

171.   Always be gentle when giving someone else a message. Even if the person you are massaging complains, you should avoid applying too much pressure to their muscles and joints. Unless you have been trained in message therapy, you are more likely to hurt them than to relieve their pain by being more forceful.

172.   Make the most of your massage by drinking lots of water. Why? Because a good massage gets your circulation going, but water is needed to flush toxins out of your body. Hydrating before your massage makes your blood less sluggish, making it easier for the masseuse to rub excess lactic acid out of your muscles. Staying hydrated after aids your body in processing and eliminating these toxins.

173.   Be prompt to your massage so that you do not miss it. It is very easy to lose track of the time in the hustle and bustle of your day. When this happens and you find yourself rushing in for your massage, it will take longer for you to relax during the massage. Your objective is to hit the massage table relaxed.

174.   If your baby is having a difficult time sleeping, give massage a try. Massage is relaxing and easy for any parent to do. Just rest the baby on your lap and rub the back, arms, legs and neck gently. You can even use a little oil to make the massage more enjoyable.

175.   The speed of your hands is important for the kind of massage you are trying to give. If you are looking for a massage to relax your partner, go for slow strokes. If you are looking to work out tired muscles that have been over exerted, faster strokes work better.

176.   You must realize that it takes time to become a skilled masseuse. Begin by providing massages for people you know, and ask them to provide feedback. As you become more comfortable, you can branch out and practice on other people.

177.   Before you give a massage, stretch all of the areas that you are planning to use. This means that you will need to stretch your fingers, arms, neck, back and legs so that you can reduce cramps during your massage and get all areas involved. If you are providing a long massage session, stretching is imperative.

178.   The legs are very important when giving a massage. Many of the largest muscles in the body are in the legs, and these are often the most used. Be responsive to your partner when massaging their legs and try to encompass the entire muscle group. Start up high around the butt and work your way down to the ankles.

179.   Recover slowly after enjoying a massage. Hold off on immediately jumping up from the table as soon as the masseuse leaves the room. Take a moment to luxuriate in the warm, relaxed feel of your body. Open your eyes, take in your surroundings, and then slowly sit up on the edge of the table. Rest a moment before standing.

180.   Speak up. If there is an area you want your therapist to focus heavily on, let her know. For instance, you might need to tell the masseuse to apply more pressure.

181.   When you give someone a massage, don't neglect the hands and feet. These parts of the body are most sensitive and may be where the person gets the best feelings. When massaging these places, be firm and loosen up those muscles.

182.   If you enjoy working out, you should try massaging your muscles before and after exercising.

You should pummel your muscles with your fists to improve your circulation before working out and massage your muscles more gently after working out to speed up the recovery process. Make sure you stretch after massaging.

183.   If you are pregnant and getting a massage, avoid massage tables which have holes in them. This will ensure yours and the baby's comfort and prevent the stress to your lower back. Also, make sure you use plenty of pillows as additional padding in order to feel more comfortable and secure.

184.   Before beginning your massage, discuss pressure with your massage therapist. Some people like massages that are very deep with a hard intensity. Others prefer a lighter touch or even Reiki style massages where touch is not necessary. If you let your therapist know what works for you, they can adjust the massage to meet your individual needs.

185.   When you are giving a massage, the atmosphere you provide will do wonders for your partner. Try using soft music in the background to relax your partner. Diffuser oils and candles will relax your partners senses and make them feel at ease. Also using low or soft lighting will help your partner relax and get into the mood for a great massage.

186.   A proper environment is essential to a successful therapeutic back massage at home. The ideal location is in a quiet, warm and relaxed environment. If you're not doing the massage in an area like that, the person you're massaging may not be able to relax or reap all of the benefits of a therapeutic massage.

187.   As you are preparing to conduct a massage, allow soft music to play in the background. This allows the recipient to just float away. It will also help the person get rid of muscle tension. You'll be able to work out the tight muscles better and give a more effective massage.

188.   Seek to have your massages done professionally. While it may be easier to ask for one from your spouse, you are certainly risking injury. If someone is not educated in how to properly give a massage. They can easily cause a muscle to be pulled or even something far worse.

189.   Change your mindset about massage. Instead of thinking of it as a luxury, think of massage as a therapeutic approach to health. Research shows that massage can lower levels of the stress hormone cortisol, as well as lessening asthma symptoms in children. Additionally, those tension headaches are

no match for the hands of a skilled massage therapist.

190.   If your child suffers from asthma, consider massage. Massage has been proven to help breathing in asthmatic children due to the relaxing benefits it offers. A child's massage should be done with a gentle touch and only for a limited period of time. Try this in the evening and help your child to also enjoy a good night's rest.

191.   After you give a massage to someone, make sure that they take a warm bath. This will help to further the effect of the massage and soothe the muscles even more. After this person takes the bath, they will feel more refreshed and looser then they ever had in their entire life.

192.   If your child is suffering from colic, a gentle massage may alleviate some of their suffering. Slightly warm some lavender baby lotion and gently massage your infants back, legs, hands and feet. This will help relax your child making them less fussy if they are suffering from stomach cramps caused by colic.

193.   Work slowly for a soothing benefit. If you are using your thumbs to apply pressure, be careful not to put all your weight on your thumbs. This could

cause them to tire. Support your hand with your other fingers. Use your weight to avoid fatigue, too.

194.   If you tend to have a lot of tension in your muscles, but you don't like a rigorous massage, hot stone massage might be your best choice. The stones, which are smooth, are made warm and then placed onto specific areas of the body. This warms the muscles and tissues, releasing tension and pent-up energy.

195.   Shiatsu massages come from Japan and are basically like acupuncture. The only difference is that instead of needles, fingers are used. Your therapist will hit pressure points that cause the entire body to relax. Shiatsu massage is intended to increase the subject's energy level and sense of well-being.

196.   If you are a woman, don't swear off men massage therapists. Since most women are modest, they often feel uncomfortable in front of a male massage therapist. However, some women have reported that the best massage they have gotten in a long time is from a male massage therapist. Whatever your decision, don't just base it on the sex of the massage therapist.

197.   Don't be shy about speaking up during a massage. If you have a spot you want focused on, just say so. If you think more pressure is needed, talk about it; you won't get the service you want otherwise.

198.   If you enjoy working out, you should try massaging your muscles before and after exercising. You should pummel your muscles with your fists to improve your circulation before working out and massage your muscles more gently after working out to speed up the recovery process. Make sure you stretch after massaging.

199.   You do not have to remove your clothing for a massage. Many people feel uncomfortable being completely undressed, so don't be afraid to keep some clothing on if it makes you more relaxed. Your masseuse will not be offended. The goal of a massage is to relax, so stressing about clothing is counter-productive.

200.   You can massage your eyes to make your headaches go away. If you have tired eyes, you should rub your hands together until your palms get warm. Place your warm hands over your eyes and let your palms warm up your eyes. The warmth will relax the muscles located in your eyes.

201.   Remember to breathe deeply when receiving a massage. You want to bring oxygen to every part of your body to enhance the healing effects of the massaging action. Breathe in and out of your nose to create a meditative type state, and make sure to breathe deep into your abdomen.

202.   If you live to give massages, think about getting a license. The proper training to be a massage therapist is very short, and it will allow you to make a living. You can work at a clinic or build your own clientele.

203.   Prior to making your first visit to a massage clinic, make sure you research the facility. Consumers often post reviews online, and the Better Business Bureau will let you know if there have been any complaints lodged against the practice. Finally, you can also talk to your local Department of Health.

204.   Always look for online reviews before going to a massage therapist. Every spa and clinic out there probably has a review about them on the Internet. By reviewing the opinions of other people, you will be better able to select a few therapists to consider.

205.   If you are short on time or short on money, consider getting a chair massage. A chair massage

usually lasts for about 10 minutes and is much less expensive than a full body massage. A typical chair massage runs about $10 to $15 and can be easily fit into a busy schedule.

206.   Change your mindset about massage. Instead of thinking of it as a luxury, think of massage as a therapeutic approach to health. Research shows that massage can lower levels of the stress hormone cortisol, as well as lessening asthma symptoms in children. Additionally, those tension headaches are no match for the hands of a skilled massage therapist.

207.   Only disrobe to your comfort level. For many people, undressing for a massage is not a big deal. This is not the case with some and they often find themselves feeling uncomfortable or self-conscious during the massage. This will reduce the effect of the massage. Avoid this by only taking off the clothing you are comfortable with.

208.   Your massage therapist needs to be capable to get to your skin in order to do the massage, so you need to be prepared to disrobe. You will be able to do this in the room alone, and you can leave on your underwear. Once you are undressed and face down on the massage table under a sheet, then the therapist will return to the room.

209.   If you have a wound that is beginning to heal, massaging around that area will help it to heal even faster. Massage increases the amount of blood that is flowing to that area of your body. So, by massaging that area you are providing it with new blood to promote healing. This can also help to reduce scars.

210.   Do not get up immediately after your massage, especially when receiving a deep tissue massage. Most people will experience bouts of dizziness or feeling light-headed if the body has not had time to process the ministrations of the masseuse. Relax a bit more and let your body regulate itself before you get back to your day.

211.   A great place to start with a massage is the back. When you start on your partner's back, you will give their body an overall relaxation that is more conducive to massaging the rest of the body. The quicker you can get their entire body to relax, the more beneficial the entire massage will be.

212.   Newcomers to massages should go for either a Swedish massage or deep tissue massage. Lots of options exist, and some might disappoint you if you are in need of serious attention. The types mentioned above are the most popular.

213.   What should one use for a self-massage? Whatever you can use! If you're massaging a knot out of your thigh, why not use your elbow? Is your neck sore? Fingers will do, but you can also buy a massaging neck roller. Try out different items and body parts and see what works for you.

214.   Ease stomach pain and aid digestion by massaging your belly. After a big meal, try rubbing your abdomen clockwise with both hands. This procedure can help to facilitate your digestion and ease distress. Be very gentle and do not apply pressure on your abdomen until you are done digesting.

215.   Be on time, or a little early. Besides being good etiquette, being punctual can actually help your massage be effective. When you are running late, you are usually in a frenzied state, increasing stress levels and putting your body on edge. In a massage, this means it will take you longer to unwind and you may not get all of the benefits of a relaxing rub down.

216.   Aromatherapy massage uses scented therapeutic massage oils along with gentle kneading motions. These scented oils add another dimension to the standard massage by incorporating the sense of

smell into the massage therapy. Aromatherapy often uses lavender, eucalyptus and chamomile. This type of massage is perfect for people suffering for stress related pain.

217.   Wake yourself up in the morning or calm yourself down at night with a good massage! To do this, gently thump your body with your fists. Begin at your legs and arms and go from bottom to top. This massage is great for relieving stress and tension. However, avoid this massage if you are currently taking any blood thinners because you could bruise your body.

218.   Ask your therapist if he or she has a referral programs. Your massages could be low priced or free if you can refer others. A nearly-free massage is perfect when your budget is tight and you need some stress-reduction to make it through the weekend.

219.   Drink plenty of water both before and after your massage. It can be tempting to come home from your massage relaxed and ready for a nap. However, it's important to flush harmful toxins out the body, so be sure to drink water.

220.   If you have a less than pleasant experience having a massage, try not to write them off

completely. Everyone has their own style and techniques and no two massage therapists are the same. Ask for a recommendation from a friend for someone new, and explain your experience to them so they can do their best to make your massage with them as pleasant as possible.

221.   Do not immediately engage in strenuous activity following a massage. Taking a short, calming walk or sitting and reading for a few minutes would be ideal. It is often reported that people feel dizzy following a massage, and this means that the body is not ready to jump into heavy lifting or heart racing activities. It is fine to enjoy these activities a little later in the day, about an hour or so after your massage.

222.   good way to eliminate stress and pain is by getting a massage. If you have chronic back aches or have other stress related issues, you should regularly have a massage. Find someone to give you a great massage or visit a professional masseuse.

223.   If your child suffers from asthma, consider massage. Massage has been proven to help breathing in asthmatic children due to the relaxing benefits it offers. A child's massage should be done with a gentle touch and only for a limited period of

time. Try this in the evening and help your child to also enjoy a good night's rest.

224.   Make sure that your massage therapist is registered in your state. If your massage therapist is not properly registered and insured, then you are at risk of being left to fend for yourself if they were to cause injury to you during their work. Do not worry about being rude, ask for proof so that you can be confident that you are in responsible hands.

225.   Don't underestimate the value of a good massage. Getting a massage can relieve pain, eliminate stress and provide you with energy. Regardless of the kind of health issues you have, you should consider getting a massage from a professional to see for yourself.

226.   Swedish massage therapy is the most frequently offered type available. Some people consider this to just be a basic massage. The strokes are long and smooth, done in a kneading motion, typically in circles. The masseuse will normally use oil during the process. It is not too rigorous and quite enjoyable.

227.   When you're stressed out or feeling emotional, aromatherapy massage is for you. The therapist will use essential oils while massaging your skin. They

know exactly which oils will give you energy, relax you or help to bust stress. Lavender is frequently used to calm your mind and body, allowing you some peace.

228.   Don't rush to stand up following a massage. You've been lying down, completely relaxed, for a long time. You may feel lightheaded when starting to rise, so take caution.

229.   Athletes use a simple method to massage their feet. You can roll over a tennis ball or a golf ball with your feet. Just move sideways and back and forth. Concentrate on the area that is most sensitive.

230.   If you are a woman, don't swear off men massage therapists. Since most women are modest, they often feel uncomfortable in front of a male massage therapist. However, some women have reported that the best massage they have gotten in a long time is from a male massage therapist. Whatever your decision, don't just base it on the sex of the massage therapist.

231.   If you are getting a full body massage, always ask to take a shower or at least wash your feet prior to beginning the massage. You can hold a lot of dirt and bacteria on places like your feet and hands, and

you do not want your massage therapist massaging those areas first and then placing their hands on your face for further massage.

232.   Massage right to the tips of the digits on hands and feet. These are among the two most sensitive parts of the body and can cause great feelings through the entire massage. When massaging these places, be firm and loosen up those muscles.

233.   Massage can help your marriage if you have a high stress job. When you come home after a hard day at work, as soothing massage by your mate can increase your love and appreciation for him or her. Instead of feeling too tired for romance, you will be more open to spending some quality time.

234.   If you are pregnant and getting a massage, avoid massage tables which have holes in them. This will ensure yours and the baby's comfort and prevent the stress to your lower back. Also, make sure you use plenty of pillows as additional padding in order to feel more comfortable and secure.

235.   Do not forget to tip your massage therapist. Many therapists work mostly for tips and only receive a small percentage of the price you pay for the massage. They will appreciate a good tip, and it

will be remembered the next time you return. A fair tip is typically fifteen to twenty percent.

236.   Wake yourself up in the morning or calm yourself down at night with a good massage! To do this, gently thump your body with your fists. Begin at your legs and arms and go from bottom to top. This massage is great for relieving stress and tension. However, avoid this massage if you are currently taking any blood thinners because you could bruise your body.

237.   If you are giving a deep tissue massage, incorporate your elbows into it. This may feel uncomfortable at first for the person you are massaging, but is a fantastic way of spreading out the muscle and causing a very pleasurable sensation. Never push too hard though, as this will then feel uncomfortable.

238.   A great massage to relieve strained shoulders is a bear hug. To begin, cross your arms over your chest. Grab your shoulder with either hand. Then, squeeze a shoulder and release it about three times. Do this for both of them. After that, move down your arms, squeezing and releasing them until you reach your wrists.

239.   Don't make the mistake of thinking that you have to spend a lot of money to get a good massage. Meanwhile, it is human nature to choose well known spas, a smaller center or a massage school can offer the same services. Sometimes lesser known places offer better massages than their more expensive counterparts, for half the price.

240.   When providing a massage, be sure to use the thumbs. This area can elicit a great feeling on those you massage. Don't push incredibly hard since it can cause some discomfort to that person you're massaging.

241.   Start your massage at the top of the back. This is important as there are a lot of muscles and knots tied up in this area. This technique will help you to soothe the person you are massaging and serves as a great bridge to the other areas of the body.

242.   You want to be at your massage appointment a little early. You can easily be lost in time. When this occurs and you end up rushing to get to your massage on time, you won't be able to fully relax during your massage session. You must be totally relaxed when it's time to be massaged.

243.   Arthritis is a painful condition. While medication may be necessary for your situation, it

may not do as good of a job as you need it to. If medication is not working, try getting a massage. The increased circulation and flexibility encouraged by massage can help relieve arthritis pain.

244. A foot massage can be used for more than tired, achy feet. You can search online and find foot maps that show which area of the foot can be massaged to experience relief from a myriad of symptoms throughout your body. For example, pressing on the big toe is known to relieve sinus pain and pressure.

245. If your goal is to calm the massage recipient, use movements that are slow. If you move your hands too fast or generally attack the back, you'll definitely not create a relaxing atmosphere! Instead focus on being calm yourself. Slow down your pace and move slowly but deliberately. Wait for cues from the massage recipient as to whether to speed up or slow down even more.

246. Put your thinking on hold. One of the most difficult, yet essential elements of getting the most out of a massage is relaxing your mental state. Try to start doing some deep breathing while the therapist is setting up. Imagine that, with every inhale, you gather all the nagging and stressful thoughts in your head. On the exhale, envision

blowing all of these thoughts out into space, gone forever. Keep repeating until you feel yourself relaxing.

247.   If you need help with stress or pain, you should get a massage from a professional. Asking someone you know to give you a massage can be helpful but keep in mind that a trained professional will be able to use technique your friend or relative does not know about.

248.   When you get a massage, request that the lights be dimmed. A darker room is more calming and peaceful as it resembles night time. You should not make the room entirely dark, but it will be easier to relax if you are not exposed to bright lights.

249.   The art of Shiatsu massage uses fingers instead of needles in a form of massage acupuncture. Your therapist will place pressure on key areas which will prompt instant relaxation. The goal of a Shiatsu massage is to increase a person's energy level and well being.

250.   The Japanese love to engage in a form of massage called shiatsu. This uses the pressure from the masseuse's fingers pressed in a rhythm on your acupuncture meridians. The pressure is applied for a few to many seconds, boosting energy flow and

returning the body to balance. It doesn't leave you sore, either!

251.   Whenever you get yourself a massage, don't be afraid to inform your massage therapist of your problem areas. The goal of your massage is muscle relaxation where you need it most. Your therapist is probably not a mind reader, so always let them know before starting the massage where you need the most help.

252.   Use candles to set the mood. Candles provide subtle lighting, while simultaneously creating a relaxing atmosphere. Scented candles are also a great idea. Place them evenly throughout the room, at varying elevations. It is also important to be safe when using candles. Keep them away from hanging fabric such as curtains.

253.   There are a few secrets to giving a fantastic massage and they involve things you don't do. Always be careful to not pull their hair. Body hair is included in this. Be careful of pressure on their bones. Learn to be gentle when you need to be and hard when required.

254.   Be on time, or a little early. Besides being good etiquette, being punctual can actually help your massage be effective. When you are running late,

you are usually in a frenzied state, increasing stress levels and putting your body on edge. In a massage, this means it will take you longer to unwind and you may not get all of the benefits of a relaxing rub down.

255.   Eat some food about 30 minutes prior to a massage, but don't eat too much! You don't want to feel bloated for the experience. You want just enough food that you feel relaxed. If you go in hungry, you'll be that much more stressed for the entire time period of the massage.

256.   Make the most of your massage by drinking lots of water. Why? Because a good massage gets your circulation going, but water is needed to flush toxins out of your body. Hydrating before your massage makes your blood less sluggish, making it easier for the masseuse to rub excess lactic acid out of your muscles. Staying hydrated after aids your body in processing and eliminating these toxins.

257.   Before you begin a massage, put a drop of the oil you are planning to use on the client and let it sit for a moment to avoid allergic reactions. This will enable you to ensure that they are not allergic or will not have a reaction to that specific oil. It is important to apply oil because it provides

lubrication at the points of contact and make you feel better.

258.   You can make massages even better by using some massaging oils. There are plenty of different essential oils to choose from. Choose an oil with an enjoyable smell and you will find that massages are even more relaxing thanks to the smell of the essential oils and the properties of the oil you chose.

259.   A foot massage can be used for more than tired, achy feet. You can search online and find foot maps that show which area of the foot can be massaged to experience relief from a myriad of symptoms throughout your body. For example, pressing on the big toe is known to relieve sinus pain and pressure.

260.   If you will be getting a massage to have some stress relieved, go with an aromatherapy massage. Along with a massage, the therapist will use essential oils on your capillaries in order to relax the body. Most of these oils come from flowers, roots, and herbs and are completely safe.

261.   When you decide to get a massage, make sure you are communicating with your massage therapist. If you have any massage preferences, make sure you tell him or her when entering the

room and before starting. If during the massage you are feeling pain or experiencing numbness, make sure you let your therapist know by speaking up.

262.   When you are giving a massage, a quiet environment is desirable. The worst thing in the world is to try to unwind and relax, only to have your masseuse talk your ear off. Music is the only sound one should hear. Beyond that, you want to operate in silence.

263.   It is important to share any problem areas you are having with your massage therapist. The goal is to relax the muscles and address your issue areas. Remember that your massage therapist will not know about problem areas unless you tell them.

264.   You need to clean your feet before getting a good full body massage. Your feet may carry lots of fungus and bacteria that your masseuse can easily spread during a complete body massage when working the body. Staying clean will help you feel refreshed and relaxed during your massage.

265.   If you're always catching an illness from everyone else, there is some hope! Massage boosts white blood cell production. They are a key point of your immune system to help you fight illness.

266.   Before beginning your massage, discuss pressure with your massage therapist. Some people like massages that are very deep with a hard intensity. Others prefer a lighter touch or even Reiki style massages where touch is not necessary. If you let your therapist know what works for you, they can adjust the massage to meet your individual needs.

267.   If you are battling cancer it can really take a toll on your body. You are probably feeling a little depressed, some anxiety, fatigue and nausea from the treatments and the diagnosis in general. Having a massage has been proven to help fight off all of these symptoms, which can help you to fight even that much harder to beat it.

268.   When you are going for a massage, make sure that you communicate with your therapist. Going to a massage therapist is similar to going to a doctor. Have any questions or concerns ready when you go to the appointment. Tell the therapist about any areas that need work, the type of massage you would like or ask any questions about different kinds of massages you may have heard about.

269.   Shiatsu massage is used by gently applying firm pressure into affected meridians then quickly releasing it. This type of massage is perfect for those suffering from tired muscles that need

immediate relief. Unlike other types of massage, this massage does not leave the person feeling sore afterwards; instead, they feel refreshed and renewed.

270. If you are thinking about finding a massage therapist, ask your doctor for a recommendation. Often, your doctor will be able to refer you to an excellent professional from their years of experience in dealing with health problems. You might also ask a trainer at your gym to refer you to an excellent massage therapist.

271. Massaging is a great way to relieve pain and stress but keep in mind that a massage might not be your best option if your joints or articulations are bothering you. You should go to a chiropractor for some adjustments instead of massaging or trying to adjust your joints yourself.

272. You should massage your hands when you plan to moisturize the rest of your body. Start by putting your fingers together so that your palms are touching and rub them together in a circular fashion. Next, massage below your thumb in a circular motion. Use your index fingers and thumbs to massage the wrists, palms and fingers.

273. Massage tools are a great addition to the traditional massage. You can make massages much

more efficient by using accessories such as massage balls. Affordable massage tools can be found in stores or online. Try each of the tools that you can find and see which ones fit your program.

274.   If you are an athlete or have excessively hard workouts then having massages regularly is a good idea. Massages can loosen your muscles up before a game or exercise to help them from becoming injured. It can also help after strenuous exercise to help heal your muscles and keep them from stiffening up or becoming painful.

275.   If you have problems with tension headaches and medication is not doing the trick, consider massage. Massage helps to relax the body, and it can target specific pressure points that offer benefits. Enjoying a massage once a week might be all you need to get rid of your headaches and keep them away.

276.   A popular back massage you can try out on someone is called a "Raking Massage". With this technique, you spread your fingers apart and use your tips to give the massage. Begin in the shoulder area and work your way down the back using a raking motion. Then, you move your fingers down the spine without actually touching it. Move one hand down as the other hand moves up.

277.   When using massage oil, before putting it on a person's back, place it into your hands first. If you place the oil directly onto your partner, the oil may be surprisingly cold and startle the person. That's not the kind of reaction you want from a massage. Instead place the oil first in your hands and warm the oil up by rubbing your hands together. This will make the oil the perfect temperature to use.

278.   If you tend to have a lot of tension in your muscles, but you don't like a rigorous massage, hot stone massage might be your best choice. The stones, which are smooth, are made warm and then placed onto specific areas of the body. This warms the muscles and tissues, releasing tension and pent-up energy.

279.   Do not hesitate to talk to your doctor about massages. If you deal with back pains or muscle pains on a regular basis, ask your doctor if massages would be a good solution. Your doctor should be able to recommend a good massage clinic in your area and even write you a prescription.

280.   If you are getting a full body massage, always ask to take a shower or at least wash your feet prior to beginning the massage. You can hold a lot of dirt and bacteria on places like your feet and hands, and

you do not want your massage therapist massaging those areas first and then placing their hands on your face for further massage.

281.   Be on time for the massage. While it's time to relax, it doesn't mean you come in late. The massage therapists are on a schedule and have to attend to other clients as well, so don't keep them waiting.

282.   If you are battling cancer it can really take a toll on your body. You are probably feeling a little depressed, some anxiety, fatigue and nausea from the treatments and the diagnosis in general. Having a massage has been proven to help fight off all of these symptoms, which can help you to fight even that much harder to beat it.

283.   When giving a massage, remember to relax yourself. If you are holding a lot of tension, it will be more difficult to maneuver your hands in a way that provides a great massage. The tension will also show through in your attention to each area of the body and the overall feel of the room.

284.   Try not to go to a massage appointment with a full stomach. It is better to have eaten about half an hour before your appointment. A massage requires that you lay on your stomach for an extended

period of time, and this can be very uncomfortable if your belly is too full.

285.   Avoid eating before a massage. You want at least 90 minutes between your last meal and your massage. However, more time is better. Allow your body to digest its meal so you can fully relax and get all the benefits of your massage. As a bonus you will be spared embarrassing stomach gurgling noises during your session.

286.   When you are giving a massage, the atmosphere you provide will do wonders for your partner. Try using soft music in the background to relax your partner. Diffuser oils and candles will relax your partners senses and make them feel at ease. Also using low or soft lighting will help your partner relax and get into the mood for a great massage.

287.   Look into getting massages from students if you are on a slim budget. Massages can be very expensive, but students are always looking for people to practice on and they are usually very good. Additionally, their teacher is on hand for advice, so you are usually in really good hands.

288.   If you often experience back pain, you should consider investing in a vibrating massaging pad. Some pads even have an option that allows you to

apply heat to your muscles. Compare different products before you purchase on and choose one with different speeds so you can easily adjust it in function of your needs.

289.   Make sure you aren't holding your breath during your massage session. Pressure massage is important to work out the kinks and pains in your muscles. The stored up pension cannot be eliminated if you are holding your breath the whole time. If you are feeling nervous, try some deep and slow breathing exercises before starting your session.

290.   Hydrate yourself well for forty-eight hours before your massage. Many people know that heavy water intake after a massage is good for flushing the body of toxins and helping with sore muscles. Drinking plenty of water before the massage will greatly increase the impact of the massage and its purging abilities.

291.   If a person wants a deeper massage, be careful on how much oil, you use. Yes, oil feels great on a person's back and causes less friction, but the latter is the problem for deeper tissue massage. Without that friction, you won't be able to offer a deep massage, as your hands will constantly slide. Minimize this issue by using just enough oil for the

massage to be comfortable, but not so much that you lose all friction.

292.   If your child is suffering from colic, a gentle massage may alleviate some of their suffering. Slightly warm some lavender baby lotion and gently massage your infants back, legs, hands and feet. This will help relax your child making them less fussy if they are suffering from stomach cramps caused by colic.

293.   Help the massage therapist by relaxing your body. Avoid trying to "help" by tensing certain muscles or areas. The massage therapist is well-educated in various ways to maneuver your body parts to achieve the best results from massage, but their work is hindered if you can't relax. Try doing some deep breathing and practice just letting go and trusting the therapist to do a great job.

294.   When you are giving massages, try to be quiet. When you want to unwind and relax on the massage table, nothing is more annoying than having the masseuse talk and talk. Nature sound or quiet music should be the sole sound. Besides that, things should be very quiet.

295.   Have you been having trouble sleeping at night? This is a common problem that a lot of people have

in common. If you are leery about taking prescription or over the counter sleep aids, there is a solution. Having a massage relaxes you mind, body and spirit, which helps you to fall asleep easier each night.

296. Talk to your massage therapist about your health issues before the massage. This would include any information about a pregnancy. This information will assist the massage therapist in tailoring the massage to your specific needs. You massage therapist will be ill-equipped to help you if you don't disclose all.

297. Massage is an important part of spending time at a luxury spa. Although most people cannot afford this type of indulgence on a regular basis, visiting a spa a few times during the year can provide the type of rejuvenation everyone needs from time to time. Enjoy the massage and every other part of your day to the fullest.

298. There is a helpful massage that helps to relieve sinus pressure and congestion. To do this massage, begin by placing your fingers right above your nose and pressing down. Be sure you are rubbing outward. Next, put your fingers under your eyes, moving down and rubbing out. Massage the

cheekbones with your thumbs and then put your thumbs on your temples, moving in small circles.

299.   You should ask for feedback when giving a massage to someone. Remind the person that you have no way of knowing how efficient your massage is if they do not let you know how they feel. Encourage the person to guide you so you can find the area that is tense.

300.   Be sure to give massages in a relaxed environment. Massage is all about releasing tension and relaxing. An environment filled with noise can be stressful and not relaxing. It should be so peaceful that the client might even doze off. Use quiet music and turn down the lights to achieve that serene effect.

301.   If you have a less than pleasant experience having a massage, try not to write them off completely. Everyone has their own style and techniques and no two massage therapists are the same. Ask for a recommendation from a friend for someone new, and explain your experience to them so they can do their best to make your massage with them as pleasant as possible.

302.   One great massage technique that you can do for your partner is called raking. Raking means that

you spread your hands out, and using your fingertips, you rake up one side of the back right by the spine while you rake downward on the other side with your other hand.

303.   Always be gentle when giving someone else a message. Even if the person you are massaging complains, you should avoid applying too much pressure to their muscles and joints. Unless you have been trained in message therapy, you are more likely to hurt them than to relieve their pain by being more forceful.

304.   When giving a massage, do not forget to focus some attention on the neck and shoulders. While much attention is paid to the back during a massage, the neck and shoulders can hold tension and stress too. Spending some time massaging them offers a lot of relief and can improve the massage experience.

305.   One simple way to give a massage is to use a "raking" technique. This is done by spreading your fingers and using your fingertips. Start in the shoulder area then move your fingers in a raking motion down the back. Make sure the fingers move along the spine not on top of the spine. While one hand moves up move the other one down in alternating motion.

306.   When giving a massage, it is very important that you use oil or lotion. Massage oils can increase the movements of the soft tissue. Using oil will minimize the pinching and tugging feel on the skin. Massage oils come in all different varieties. They include aromatherapy and provide lubrication and nutrients.

307.   When you are giving a massage, try not to use the same stroke over and over. This can make the whole experience mundane, as you want to incorporate as much change during the session as possible. Alter your technique, the stroke and how hard you press on the back, neck and thighs.

308.   Asian massages are known to help relax the body. One not-so-common, but very relaxing Asian massage is called the Indonesian-Javanese massage. With this method, the therapist will use both their hands and knuckles to get so deep into the skin. This will help your muscles relax if they were tense.

309.   When massaging someone, open your fingers up so that you can be more precise with the area that you massage. This helps to loosen up the muscles and is also a great technique if you are planning on giving a deep tissue massage. After you massage this way, close your hands back up and use your palms.

310.   Before you give a massage, stretch all of the areas that you are planning to use. This means that you will need to stretch your fingers, arms, neck, back and legs so that you can reduce cramps during your massage and get all areas involved. If you are providing a long massage session, stretching is imperative.

311.   If you're pregnant, you can still enjoy a massage if it is given by a license therapist. This is a great way to deal with morning sickness, stress, back pain, sore breasts and swollen ankles. You can continue it after birth to deal with postpartum depression, weight loss and baby-carrying pains, too.

312.   When you have a client that you are giving a massage to, ask whether or not they are comfortable. The last thing that you will want is someone who does not feel secure when you are giving a massage. Additionally, they will be very tight and tough to massage if they are anxious.

313.   Recover slowly after enjoying a massage. Hold off on immediately jumping up from the table as soon as the masseuse leaves the room. Take a moment to luxuriate in the warm, relaxed feel of your body. Open your eyes, take in your

surroundings, and then slowly sit up on the edge of the table. Rest a moment before standing.

314.   It is important to feel free to ask for any specific requests you have for your masseuse., Let your masseuse know what areas you'd like them to focus on. If you need more intensity in some areas to work out the kinks, then you need to speak up so the masseuse will know.

315.   Massage is an important part of spending time at a luxury spa. Although most people cannot afford this type of indulgence on a regular basis, visiting a spa a few times during the year can provide the type of rejuvenation everyone needs from time to time. Enjoy the massage and every other part of your day to the fullest.

316.   Take advantage of the non-human massages that you can get. Instead of going to a person for your massage, there are different whirlpools that you can use, which have jets that can massage your back and body. This can be a great form of not only relief, but exercise as well.

317.   If you are on the giving end of a very beneficial massage, make sure to read the signs the recipient is showing. During a deep-tissue massage, the body responds to pressure and muscles will actually

contract under your finger-tips. Ease up on the pressure when you approach bones and joints and be guided by the response you get!

318.   If you have a less than pleasant experience having a massage, try not to write them off completely. Everyone has their own style and techniques and no two massage therapists are the same. Ask for a recommendation from a friend for someone new, and explain your experience to them so they can do their best to make your massage with them as pleasant as possible.

319.   If you suffer from frequent tension headaches, you may benefit from a professional deep tissue neck massage. To perform a deep tissue massage, the massage therapist uses a stretching technique along with pressure to pull and stretch your muscles. This allows the muscles to relax; thus, relieving your headache and tension.

320.   Do not eat before you go for a massage, as this can make you feel bloated. It'll leave you bloated and uncomfortable when lying down. Digest all of your food and have a light snack before the massage. This will let you feel more comfortable in whatever position you are asked to adopt while getting massaged.

321.   Only disrobe to your comfort level. For many people, undressing for a massage is not a big deal. This is not the case with some and they often find themselves feeling uncomfortable or self-conscious during the massage. This will reduce the effect of the massage. Avoid this by only taking off the clothing you are comfortable with.

322.   Try to limit all background noise when you are giving your massage, as the environment should be as quiet and calm as possible at all times. You will want the person you are massaging to relax their muscles so that your massage technique will work, as a quiet atmosphere helps to facilitate this.

323.   Make sure that your massage therapist is registered in your state. If your massage therapist is not properly registered and insured, then you are at risk of being left to fend for yourself if they were to cause injury to you during their work. Do not worry about being rude, ask for proof so that you can be confident that you are in responsible hands.

324.   Try using the bear hugging technique if you retain tension in your shoulders. Wrap your arms over your chest area, like making an x. Place a hand on each of your shoulders and massage. This is an easy way to get rid of tension while quickly massaging yourself, no matter what time it is.

325.   Ask for the lights to be turned down. A darkened room is more relaxing than one with bright lights, and relaxation is the point of massage. Try to make sure the ambiance is right by keeping the light similar to that created by candles.

326.   Immediately after a massage, ensure you get up very slowly. You've been lying down, completely relaxed, for a long time. You may end up dizzy and out of sorts if you stand up quickly.

327.   You can give yourself a hand massage by using a pencil with an eraser. Use the pencil eraser to press into the fleshy areas of your hand, paying particular attention to the thumb pad. Move the eraser in a circular motion around your hand maximizing the pressure if it is necessary.

328.   Finding the right therapist is very important when it comes to massages. You do not want to visit an inexperienced or inept therapist who may cause you more harm than good. Ask friends or family if they know of a good one in your area or look on the Internet for reviews.

329.   Massage is an important part of spending time at a luxury spa. Although most people cannot afford this type of indulgence on a regular basis, visiting a

spa a few times during the year can provide the type of rejuvenation everyone needs from time to time. Enjoy the massage and every other part of your day to the fullest.

330.   When getting a massage, you need to fully relax as the therapist moves your body and joints. You do not need to try to help the therapist move your limbs and body. Think of it as being a puppet, with the therapist moving your body as they want and you just along for the ride.

331.   If you are getting a massage and you do not feel comfortable or suddenly feel like you are in pain, do not be afraid to end it. You are the paying customer whose pleasure should be the number one concern, so if you feel discomfort at any time, you have the right to conclude your session.

332.   Do not immediately engage in strenuous activity following a massage. Taking a short, calming walk or sitting and reading for a few minutes would be ideal. It is often reported that people feel dizzy following a massage, and this means that the body is not ready to jump into heavy lifting or heart racing activities. It is fine to enjoy these activities a little later in the day, about an hour or so after your massage.

333.   Go online for help in selecting a massage therapist. If that doesn't work, talk to your primary care physician. You can also talk to a nurse or a chiropractor in the area whose work you respect. Professional recommendations are almost as good (if not better) than personal recommendations, particularly if you trust the individual.

334.   Drink plenty of water before and after your massage. Drinking before your massage session ensures that your muscles are well-hydrated and supple, making the massage more effective. Water after your massage will flush out the toxins that were released and can even help prevent soreness by hastening muscle recovery time.

335.   If you are suffering from tension in the lower muscles of your body, get a deep tissue massage. There are five muscle layers in your body as this massage gets the lowest level of muscles. This is great if you play sports or have chronic tension that is not going away anytime soon.